Exclusive Glow

Discover The New You

Barbara Rogers

Introduction

Are you looking for natural beauty tips that won't leave you looking like you use make up? It may be hard to believe at first, but it's possible to have a skin, makeup, and hair routine in the morning that only takes minutes. Without taking much time and without spending a lot of money I'll give you some ideas to look your best.

What this book covers:

Ensuring your skin coloring is spot on is the first hurdle you'll need to go over to get an organic look. In some cases, you may need to seek the expert guidance of a dermatologist, but another way that works for most people is to get the help of the makeup experts working in a mall near you. I'm sure some of your friends always look great, asking them what items they use is a great way to get an idea of where to start. Another important thing to get the best look for you is to try lots of different products, and you can get free samples from many cosmetics salespeople in malls. You can also get samples of free cosmetic products online.

Reducing the amount of products you use to get ready for your day is another great way to get a more organic look. A terrific way to start limiting your product usage is to pick 3-5 different makeup products that you need every day and to try to get ready using just those products. With only three different products like lip gloss, mascara, and concealer you can achieve a fantastic look. In only a few minutes, I can have my makeup finished and be heading for work.

If you're one of the women out there who use loads of products every morning and have wanted to start looking more natural, don't change everything all at once. By just removing one or two cosmetics from your normal routine you'll see that you don't really need all those products to look great.

The foundation for beauty can be challenging. One will often be happy to find the right solution as a foundation. If liquid or cream foundation leaves you feeling 'made up' there are several natural beauty tips you can try to get rid of that feeling. With a mineral powder, you can get a fantastic look, and you won't have to cake on this product to get the look you want.

That perfect look you've been fantasizing about in your head can be a reality if you take my fashion help and make it part of your routine. After you've discovered the makeup that works for you, bring out even more of your natural beauty by making intelligent life choices like sleeping well and eating a healthy diet. Thank you for choosing to read this book. I am sure it will be helpful in your beauty plans, read on.

Table of Contents

Chapter 1:
Natural Beauty Tips

Acne is the common problem which is faced by almost every woman along with some men. However, men are not the main focus of this book. Therefore, here are some tips for preventing acne. Some beauty tips for women to prevent acne;

1. Regularly do a washing of the face with clean water and detergent

2. Water

3. Diet

4. Cleansing and toning

5. Quick solution

Some natural beauty tips;

The best way to enhance your beauty since natural products don't have any side effects and does not cause any harm. Listed below are some natural ways by which you can embellish your beauty:-

1. Applying natural products: Natural products like curd, turmeric, milk, lemon, honey, ginger, etc. is excellent for the skin. To make skin bright and glowing, consider the application of ginger paste and honey early in the morning. Besides, one of the best remedies for tanning in turmeric paste and lemon juice with the inclusion of raw milk. This also makes the skin brighter. Washing skin with buttermilk tones your skin. For a dry skin mixture of honey and lemon can be applied.

2. Healthy Diet: Eating healthy makes skin look clean and clear. Fruits such as bananas are an anti-aging agent. Oranges are key to help in making skin look tighter and also firmer. It also as anti-blemishing action. Papaya helps in the regeneration of dead cells of the skin. Oranges also have a fight against anti-aging. Water also plays an important role. It helps in maintaining the balance, for the oil generating glands. This is achieved by controlling the PH of the body.

Some valuable tips to help boost up your beauty;

1. Face pack: by the application of face pack, one can restore much of the oil in the body. It helps in removing dirt, excess oil and dead skill from the skin.

2. Good amount of sleep: Sleep about 6-8 hours help in having glowing skin, an insufficient amount of sleep makes skin look pale wan and yellowish.

3. Lip tip: If you have cracked lips, you should apply lip balm or lip gloss which can repair your lips and can give you a glossy tinge.

4. Lotion: Lotion makes the skin smoother. It also keeps the skin moisturized. You should also apply sunscreen lotion before going in the sun.

The most effective natural beauty tips are those that have an effect as speedy as possible, and this isn't limited to just products, it can also include good solid advice. Some of the most solid are centered on the way a woman engages in talking about herself internally and her perception of herself. Some good advice too is to learn self-acceptance and the knowledge that everyone is gorgeous. The reality is that these things can start changing right away in a woman's life.

One of the natural beauty tips considered to be the simplest is the utilization of positive self-talk. This begins with using affirming language; instead of talking in negative ways about yourself. You might wonder if this is a way to improve one's external beauty, but the truth is, it can because being positive on the inside shows on the outside. These subtle clues that are given indicate to others that you believe in yourself and others should too.

There are other things to do that are good pieces of advice, including that the happiest people are those who just be who they are. This can be a challenge, but once achieved it can alter your whole perception of your appearance. When you change the way you see yourself to the real you, you are almost guaranteed to view everything in a new way. This will also allow you to impact your life positively and how others see you too.

One of the ways to instantly feel uplifted is simple and straight forward. Just wear clothes that you are comfortable with and feel great while in them. When thinking about choices of styles suiting women who are 40, and above this can include making changes to the wardrobe that eliminate things that you don't like to wear. To achieve the best results possible, these first steps can help women find the clothing and styles that make them feel at their level best. It's also critical to take care of your body so that you feel confident and positive.

Taking the time to learn ways to talk both externally and internally in a manner that acknowledges your beauty is a real step to improving your life. All combined, everything here can make a woman believe in her beauty.

Chapter 2:
Beauty Through The Ages

In her lifetime, the average woman would have used cosmetics and chemical skin creams at least once in her life. And our skin is like a sponge and will almost always absorb this element sin a matter of minutes. Imagine hundreds and hundreds of these chemicals are being coursed through your veins and your body; is it doing you harm or good? Natural beauty is a gift, and it needs to be preserved and protected using natural ingredients, and nature has provided us with many of these to do that. So forget about these off-the-shelf chemicals and delve into the magical world of plants and flowers which have the power to give you back, what time has stolen.

Lesser Known Facts.

If you would have noticed, many of the skin care ads now stress on their natural ingredients. This marketing stance is taken to emphasize the points which will inspire confidence in consumers. But remember to check the fine print as well. Organic skin care Australia can provide you with a treatment plan that uses ingredients available right here in this country. Components like Manuka honey, which are only available indigenously, have so many amazing healing properties that give you exactly what you had been looking for. So stop and think before slathering on that chemical peel which boasts of fast results and switch to a more natural choice.

Real Properties from the Natural World.

If you are looking for real ingredients, then look no further than organic skin care Australia products. Their constituents include those exclusively available in the country like Manuka honey and also from places like Africa, which have unexplored lands, where plants and flowers have been known to provide their seekers a fountain of youth. Products like '100% Pure Acai Berry Anti-Ageing Eye Cream' and 'Oz Goddess Eye and Fine line cream' have used ingredients sourced from the natural world. These are what will nourish your skin and give it the power to fight its natural progression, and this is what you need to depend on.

Understanding Organic Origin.

These organic components have been available for centuries but without proper testing and extensive research, it is not possible to understand how they can be beneficial to us. Elements like strawberry, plums, cappuccino, wine and even coffee beans are everyday ingredients but their essence, which is derived from nature, is what provides some of the most amazing properties that get you results. So when you hear of deep moisturizing creams, 100% facial skin care or effective dark circle removers sourced from natural ingredients do not discount their valuable effects. Understand that these have been studied, researched and tested so as to appreciate their intrinsic properties to give you the most beneficial ones.

Eve Organics sources its ingredients from components that occur naturally both in Australia and around the world. When healthy and completely natural elements are used.

Holistic healing takes its beauty dimension from Ayurveda, which is often thought of like the other of Medicines. It considers beauty in a very different way than our more contemporary ideals of stick-thin models who pout at us from magazine covers.

The holistic healing model fits very well into the principle of the mind, the body, and the spirit of the naturally beautiful woman. Rather than only addressing the bone structure, complexion, and hip ratio of the creature, holistic beauty looks at the face as only one aspect of her appeal. In fact, we see it regarding three: the outer body, the inner body, and also the secret aspect of the girl (or boy! Ayurveda makes no distinction).

The outer body is what is perceived by the outside world, skin, bone structure, hair, nails, and teeth. To the inner body, apart from the obvious digestive processes and what might leave the body, we would also include thoughts and internal processing in general. When the inner body and the outer body work well together, the secret aspect seems to shine from the woman like the most radiant jewel.

Given this then, when the body and mind are nourished in a way that engages and galvanizes a woman, her appeal is increased one hundred fold.

Many women in our little jaunt through time were classically beautiful, but all are memorable; their incredible sense of purpose, their joy, and even when they plunged into despair to fulfill their destinies. These women are the stuff of legend, which for many of us seems entirely removed from our realities.

Any yet, we have around us just the same qualities and the same tools at our disposal to create our individual place of both greatness and serenity. Our Unforgettable Women had plants, they had gems and soils, and they had herbs. So do we. In our world of interconnectedness, we should be able to build brighter, stronger, more energetic futures than ever they did but where on earth do we start? Look in the mirror, Snow White... it has something to tell you.....

1. Consume the right things.

Consume a diet filled with whole grain products, fresh fruits, vegetables, as well as lean meats. Vegetables particularly retain the anti-oxidants your system needs to help keep your skin looking young. Make sure to reduce greasy fats and foods full of sugar.

2. Keep the skin clean.

What this means is showering, at least, one time each day and washing your face regularly, this is before going to sleep. Clean skin is freed from toxins in the environment, and of course, if you clean out the oils that the face has gathered within the day, you can prevent acne along with awful outbreaks. Stay away from the same cleanser for the body as well as your face. Additionally, make-up may clog your pores, therefore, be sure you clean it away before going to bed.

3. Make use of natural cleansers.

It is tempting to make use of the beauty products you find on television, however, that the majority of those cleansers are filled with chemicals made in a lab. Natural products are less expensive and also have no unwanted side effects. It's very rare for the natural facial cleanser, like a lemon sugar rub, to irritate the skin or even cause it to look bad. Natural skin cleansers might help your skin appear beautiful without doing harm to it.

4. Scrub the skin.

Exfoliating can help you free your skin of dead cells and clogged pores, permitting fresh, brand new skin cells to stand out. Rub your skin a bit to be able to assist exfoliating work.

5. Consume sufficient water.

The body is mainly water, which means you have to renew the cells if you would like your skin to appear beautiful. Gorgeous skin cannot be beautiful without water. Lack of fluids leads to the skin to flake and peel, and besides it tends to make new cell development slowly.

6. Get plenty of rest.

Sleep is the time our bodies regenerates itself. It is important for everyone to obtain your body the relaxation it requires so your body can perform the work of recovery. The saying "beauty sleep" truly signifies something!

Enhancing your natural beauty could be easy, even just in these hectic days. Make use of the tips outlined in this book to assist you to work on your beauty, so that you can begin looking much more gorgeous than ever before!

Chapter 3:
Skincare Solutions

Natural skin care products not only help us contribute positively to the environment, they allow us to treat our skin without applying potentially harmful chemicals to it. They are used to keep skin looking healthy, moistened, toned and radiant. While non-natural skin care products may not harm us initially, consistent use of them over time may cause more damage to our skin than they reduce. Chemical products may not just damage sensitive skin; they are known to compromise the condition of various skin types. Many people choose to produce their natural skin products at home by using the various natural ingredients available to them, but it's easy to source natural creams and ointments from a wide array of reputable and eco-friendly companies too.

Natural beauty

Most natural skin care products are comprised of 100% natural ingredients, although some have small amounts of preservatives in. Aloe Vera is categorized as one of the most useful ingredients. It is found in natural skin care products and is known widely for its positive properties. When products containing Aloe Vera are used, pleasing results can be noticed within a few weeks or so. The skin absorbs organic ingredients quicker than unnatural alternatives may. Chemical alternatives may also remove the natural oils from the skin that are so important in keeping it healthy. The essential oils that you'll tend to find in natural skin products are known for reducing stress levels as well as improving the appearance and texture of skin.

Great skin for a lifetime

Some people have different needs when it comes to skincare, and while some products are designed to appeal to those of all ages, certain products may be more beneficial when it comes to treated aging of the skin or acne for instance. The skin starts to begin the aging process from as early as five years old, but treating your skin with respect can help you to maintain a youthful appearance for longer. It's even possible to acquire skincare products for babies to promote healthy skin from the onset of life. If you're hoping to maintain a youthful appearance while sidestepping the potential damage of chemical-based products, it may well seem highly advisable to invest in natural skin care products.

It pays to take good care of the skin. This is because after all, you only have one set of it, and it has to last you a lifetime. Of course, it will age over that time, even though the body is constantly renewing the skin and that aging process will change the appearance of skin over time. To keep skin looking healthy, and as young as possible, many people opt to use skin care products and may even undergo a series of skin improvement treatments.

It is an approach that does make a lot of sense in that we humans are just part of nature, so we are at heart fed and watered by our cousins in the plant and animal kingdoms. There is also the idea that there is a wealth of cosmetics that have been known to mankind all over the world and throughout history, and that the successful ones have stayed with us whereas the, shall we say, less successful ones have not (such as the perfectly natural lead makeup that also probably killed thousands of our Roman and Elizabethan ancestors).

Horror stories aside, it is fair to say that nature has given us more than a dressing table's worth of cosmetics, from moisturizers to dyes, balms to cleansers. All that has changed is that nowadays they are packaged and ready to use, rather than being the reward for a day's walk through the jungle (although some boyfriends and husbands might still identify with that part of it). Natural skin care is also synonymous with organic skin care, a brand of the cosmetics industry that derives its ingredients from stringently natural plant extracts, right down to the fertilizers they are grown with if they are indeed commercially farmed. The words natural and organic are often used interchangeably.

Typically, naturally derived cosmetics also come with a story. The history of the cosmetic product will be told in detail, along with the way it was discovered by Western travelers and how it transformed their lives, or how the womenfolk of the tribe never seemed to age. Such tales are a fun part of the mythology behind the products and should be treated as such. The womenfolk probably did not sit next to a computer screen eight hours a day in between pollution-heavy commutes, either; but those details are often not mentioned. And besides, the proof of the pudding is in the eating. If a product does what it says it does, who cares if the marketing department has gone to town a little to paint such a romantic picture?

In the overall scheme of things, appearing in the shops might be a tiny part of the story of the magnificent, often seemingly miraculous beauty products that nature has given us. They may have been the staple of people in some global community for millennia, and will probably remain there even if the taste for natural cosmetics fades from western tastes. But on current trends, that doesn't seem likely to happen anytime soon.

For us to look our best, we take a lot of time, expend a lot of effort and spend a lot of money on our clothes, hair care products, and even our skin care products. For us to get the most value for our money, our shoes are all made from good quality leather, our clothes are from quality cotton and silks, and our skin care products are filled with lots of chemicals. Is it finally time to get some natural skin care tips?

Even though commercial after commercial on TV and ads in magazines would have us think the products we are using are fine, all of those chemicals, especially when used in conjunction with other chemicals in make-up and cleansers may not be good for your skin at all. While skin care product manufacturers that use these chemicals may test their products to ensure they don't irritate or damage our skin, they usually don't test them in conjunction with chemicals used in other products that get applied to our skin as well.

Although mixing these chemicals may not have the same effects they had in the movie, the damage they cause can be severe. Drying out the skin, possibly causing rashes and accelerating the aging process. These are some of the problems that can be caused. The only alternative is to use all natural skin care products which not only are good for our skin but in no way can harm us. Being able to use all natural products is a much healthier way to take good care of the skin.

If you read any top natural beauty blog, you see that regardless of what products you need, whether its cleansers, moisturizers, makeup removers, deep cleansing masks or anti-aging lotions, you'll be able to find everything you need to take care of the skin with all natural products. This means it doesn't matter what your skin care regimen is; you'll be able to replace all of your chemical based products with ones that are all natural. This gives you an opportunity to enjoy the benefits of beautiful skin while protecting it from the damage caused by not using natural skin care products.

Chapter 4:
Essential Beauty Oils

In aromatherapy blending, it's the essential oils that get all the press. But certain carrier oils have a very profound therapeutic activity for healing all sorts of skin conditions, as well as for daily beauty care treatment. It seems that some of the carrier oils from faraway places have the most dramatic therapeutic potential. Here're three great carrier oils from faraway places you can use alone or blend in your skin recipes that are sure to give you the healing effects you're looking for.

Our first exotic oil is pressed from rosehips seeds. These seeds grow in the mountains of South America. While these probably are very common of our "exotic" carrier oils, many people are still a little vague about its origins. Rosehips are rose flower fruit and in this case, the fruit of roses that, until recently, grew wild in a tough, mountainous environment. These small, red, round fruits are full of antioxidants (there is a pure rosehip oil available as a CO_2 extract, also excellent for skin care), and the seeds have an exceptionally fatty acid profile.

Tamanu nut oil, also called Foraha, and even sometimes Callophylum monophylum, is pressed from the nut of trees growing in tropical regions around the Pacific (specifically the islands of Vanuatu). The oil is unique in its consistency and color: the unfiltered oil is exceptionally thick and grainy, and can be solid at room temperature. The filtered oil is often still quite thick and grainy, with a dark green or brown color and somewhat pungent aroma. The grains are simply natural variations. There are variations in the makeup of the fatty acids within the oil, and will disappear when the oil is blended or applied to the skin.

Tamanu is categorized among the few "fixed" oils. It strikes a balance between a carrier oil and essential oil, possibly due to its profound therapeutic action. The oil is thought to help nearly every conceivable skin care condition. From daily moisturizing to preventing damage after exposure to sun, stimulating cellular turnover (and hence helping both wrinkles and scars), to helping the skin fight off fungal infections. The oil IS unique in appearance and smell, so you may want to blend it with other oils -- though it can be used at 100% if so desired.

Recently, Argan nut oil has been getting a lot of "press". It has been supported by the fashion and cosmetic industry, not only for its therapeutic actions, but because its production is effectively supporting indigenous people's livelihood. Further, large amounts of land have been protected so that this wonderful natural resource continues to be available.

Argan nut oil is known for its relatively high amount of natural vitamin E, along with other polyphenol antioxidants. Polyphenols are highly effective antioxidants which have other important health effects as well. Consider that it's the polyphenol "resveratrol" in red wine that has been found to extend the lifespan of many animals. Along with these micro-nutrients, Argan is full of essential fatty acids -- and the combination of these nutrients works together to create an oil with excellent anti-aging therapeutics.

If you're wanting to go all out in creating a formula, these oils can all be combined for your base mixture. Use equal parts of each -- and consider blending with a fourth oil such as coconut, evening primrose oil, apricot kernel (as you'll commonly find each of these oils recommended at twenty percent of the base oil recipe). Once you've got your base mixed, choose three essential oils to suit your skin's needs, and add seven drops of each per ounce of carrier oil blend. You'll have a truly superior skin care preparation, perfectly tailored to your skin's nee

How to reap the benefits of essential oils to treat our dry, oily, aging, wrinkly and even acne-prone facial skin:

While we may use many creams and lotions in themselves to treat our faces, essential oils are also an ancient tradition that can help our various skin types. However, it's hard to know which essential oils to use for what, and how to apply them. Straight from the bottle? Mixed or diluted with something else? The answer is quite simple. Essential oils are very strong, so the easiest ways to start reaping them when it comes to your face are:

1. By simply adding to your current moisturizer a few drops.

   Then apply it as usual (makes a great scent too!)

2. Adding facial steams to your weekly beauty care routine.

This involves hovering your head over a bowl of steaming water in which you have diluted a few drops of essential oil. You'll need a towel for this method as well to hang over your head so that it can trap in the steam, which you want to get into your pores to open them up, start to soak up the healing properties of these oils. Remember, be careful not to burn yourself!

The following are ten essential oils that will reduce the signs of aging, help fight acne and leave your face glowing with beautiful skin.

1. Lavender: Well known as a first aid remedy for burns and wounds, this oil will also help acne and scarring. Lavender oil can be applied directly to a wound, in this case, acne, to promote it's healing and prevent it from scarring by not letting it get over dry.

2. Lemon: This astringent and antiseptic make it great for treating oily skin and acne. Fresh lemons can also help get rid of acne spots by lightening the skin.

3. Rosewood: This essential oil has soothing properties, is anti-inflammatory and is ideal for relieving hot, dry, irritated skin. Because of its regenerative properties, it can be used to heal scars and treat wrinkles.

4. Neroli: This provides healing for dry, mature skin and wrinkles and may prevent stretch marks.

5. Lemongrass: A cleansing and slightly astringent substance, use in the treatment of acne and to help unblock pores.

6. Frankincense: An important rejuvenating oil that will help aging skin and wrinkles, improve skin tone and reduce scar tissue.

7. Myrrh: This Mediterranean resin from desert trees has been used in ancient times by Egyptians in many healing compounds and acts as a natural astringent. For your face, it will delay wrinkles and other visible signs of aging, which happens when our body cells start to break down.

8. Palmarosa: By stimulating cell regeneration this essential oil will improve the look of tired, aging skin

because of its balancing action and can be used for both dry and oily skin types.

9. Patchouli: This is healing and will improve the look of scars and stretch marks while also reducing wrinkles.

10. Rose: Known for being a romantic flower, in essential oil form, it is also rejuvenating and anti-inflammatory. This essential oil will help dry, irritated skin.

The bonus to using these oils as part of your beauty routine is that they also improve other areas of your general well-being. By bringing essential oils into your life, you are not only healing your skin, but also helping your bodily functions, which includes peace of mind.

Chapter 5:
Beauty Herbs For Anti-aging

Even though there are no proofs that gyno stemma is an effective herb, subsequent studies conducted in China where it originates from have come to the conclusion that once used by older people it can help give their skin a younger look as well as protect it from diseases like cancer. This natural anti-aging herb is effective when used on a regular basis as it can enhance the general functioning of your immune system thus helps to maintain the skin healthy and natural. Rhodiola, on the other hand, is one of the latest herbs discovered to be an anti-aging agent. It keeps the skin young by shielding it from excessive and direct heat mostly from the sun and once used can prohibit the development and growth of harmful cells in the body that can cause dangerous skin diseases. The Chinese wolfberry fruit provides for one of the best anti-aging herbs to protect the skin from growing old. It is most helpful in maintaining strong body muscles as well as bones and cutting down of excess weight to ensure you live longer. It is one of the herbs that apart from keeping your skin natural, soft and healthy it ensures no effects of old age affects your physical looks.

Many natural anti-aging herbs ensure one is young and stays alive for long when they are used on a regular basis. A good example of such herb is Ganoderma which has been proven over the years that it is capable of rejuvenating the respiratory and nervous systems of older people and make them function like those of young people. This is in addition to improving the immunity levels and other factors that directly influence the aging process in human beings. Likewise, acanthopanacissenticosi is another natural anti-aging herb that helps to keep one young and resistant to aging factors by reducing fatigue as well as appropriately adjusting the body system. Pseudo-Ginseng is specifically designed to handle all diseases related to the cardiovascular through taking control of how the heart functions and increasing the capacity of the major blood vessels. This ranks it as one of the most effective anti-aging herbs one can get.

Wolfberry often seen in Chinese medicine can improve the look and quality of your skin. It is a popular herb to slow down the signs of aging. Wolfberry can also treat other ailments such as insomnia, headaches, kidney disorders and eye problems.

The wolfberry also contains many other nutrients such as protein, trace minerals, Vitamin C and amino acids. It also contains antioxidants which reduce the number of fine lines on the face and body. The Siberian root which is a common use herb can also lower your stress levels as well as reduce premature aging.

Anti-aging herbs such as Goji berries has also been used in Chinese Medicine for quite some time now, and it can boost your immune system and also improve your overall health.

Be aware that not all herbs have positive effects on people, one that is commonly taken by women is the red clover. It can help reduce menstrual pain and symptoms of menopause. If taken regularly, it can minimize fine lines and wrinkles giving you a youthful-looking appearance.

When buying red clover, it can be easily found at any health food store and is usually made as an herbal supplement. Another herbal ingredient such as Aloe Vera has also been shown to improve the look of your skin as well as treat any cuts or burns on the skin. You can easily find that many products out in the market today contain aloe vera as it is very soothing to the skin.

If you are a regular sufferer of acne, using anti-aging herbs can effectively reduce your symptoms. The best three herbs that you may want to try are basil, turmeric, and mint. These herbs have an anti-bacterial and also antiseptic properties that can treat acne naturally.

Safron, which can be found in the United States, India, and the Middle East, is also used quite regularly to improve the look of your skin. To make a face mask try adding a few strands and almonds in a small amount of milk. You can then grind it and add a little amount of rose water. This will give a refreshing and cool feeling to the skin. By using these types of anti-aging herbs, you will help your skin have a better complexion as well as have smoother skin.

Please leave a review for this book. This is to help me as the author knows to what extend this writing has impacted on you as the reader.

Chapter 6:
Haircare Solutions

It is very important to take proper care of your hair if you wish to have the best personal appearance. This too demonstrates that an individual is keeping up with emerging fashion trends and hairstyles. Proper hair hygiene also ensures that your hair grows strong and healthy. Appropriate dieting will reduce cases of serious hair loss and hair breakage typically attributable to dandruff and other hair disorders related to poor dieting.

Vitamin and mineral deficiency in most cases are the main factors connected with early graying, balding and thinning of hair. Lifestyle and diet are the two major factors to be considered when choosing proper and healthy hair care procedures.

The following are a handful of the key hair care tips:

- Trimming the hair every month.

It is recommended to chop a good eighth of the hair ends so as to eliminate dead ends as well as promote faster growth of the hair.

- Brushing the hair 3-4 times to stimulate the scalp.

Stimulation of the Scalp is essential. It promotes natural oils and eradicates dead scalp cells. This is especially important for individuals suffering from dandruff. Therefore, use a high-quality hair brush to lessen hair damage cases.

- Drying hair with minimal heat.

Extreme heat in most cases will damage the hair and. Therefore, you should reduce the intensity of heat from hair curling and straightening equipment. This includes curling irons, flat irons, and blow-dryers which may damage the hair if heat frequency or intensity is not properly controlled.

- Changing hair beauty treatments.

It is advisable to substitute brushing using a wide toothed comb for detangling hot hair. It is important to use combs or brushes with smooth tips and widely spaced bristles. Combs with a sharp tooth, commonly damage the hair. They rub the scalp and lead to split ends.

- Go for the use of natural hair care products.

For example lemon, shiksa kai, coconut oil, and vinegar. It is beneficial to rinse and dry hair in lemon juice as a means of retaining shine. The issue of frizzy and tangled hair is solved by employing honey on the scalp.

- Healthy lifestyle.

This is also essential for healthy hair growth. You should start exercising regularly and avoid poor lifestyle habits which include excessive consumption of alcohol, smoking, and excessive stress.

- Wetting hair before swimming.

Wetting hair before going swimming to a beach or a pool reduces the possibility of hair soaking up chlorinated water which may be harmful to the hair. It is also highly recommended to put on a cap to protect hair from the effects of chlorinated water.

- Avoiding hair care products containing alcohol.

These products are very likely to dry out hair and increase chances of hair thinning and breakage.

- Avoiding application of hair products directly on the scalp.

These products may clog the hair pores triggering slow hair growth.

- Using soft hair tie or coated rubber band.

This is the ideal way of securing the end of braid or ponytails to help reduce the likelihood of hair damage.

- Using hair spray to maintain finished hair designs.

This provides a soft finish and can control fly away strands.

- Using pomade sparingly to braid hair.

This is important in controlling fly away ends, eliminating static and adding a glossy sheen to curl and straighten hair.

There has been some success in making use of biotin as a hair growth supplement. These cases are typically linked to age, poor dieting or post-partum hair loss cases. Hair loss may also be a consequence of stress. Most hair loss cases have been reduced through the use of ideal biotin hair care supplements incorporating silica calcium and zinc. Well formulated biotin supplements have also been found to minimize cases of hair breakage.

In summary, the above hair care tips are essential in reducing cases of hair loss, hair breakage and age-related graying of the hair. Most individuals who have applied the above procedures to boost their hair growth have witnessed positive changes in their hair management skills.

Generally speaking, we usually purchase hair care products to enhance the health of our hair while attempting to achieve a certain look and feel. We buy products with the intention of cleaning our hair. Then we have to buy products that condition our hair because the chemicals in the shampoo we just used stripped away all the natural oils. Then we purchase styling products that further damages our hair, which may require us to use hot oils and other artificial methods to repair that damage.

Comb hair with a wide-toothed comb and fluff up lightly with your fingers. Try to keep your hair dryer under the maximum heat setting and at a distance of at least 6 inches from your hair.Then move the dryer around the head constantly. Protect the ends of your hair by bending your head and blow drying with your hair hanging down. It will also give your hair more body. Leave hair slightly damp.Since natural products do not contain many chemicals, the use of such products for your hair reduces the number of chemicals your hair is exposed to. These products do not contain harmful ingredients such as pesticides, herbicides, and other chemicals. The right kinds of natural hair care products will prove safe for your skin and will also promote hair growth. Also, these products will provide a special shine to your hair that will make it look nourished, shiny and smooth.

Some people often think that it is no longer appropriate to have highlights and instead go for a more natural color. While those who continue to have highlights tone the color down, opting for a darker tone which adds more depth to the hair. However, either way of changing our hairstyle as often as many of us do can have an impact on our hair, or it's not always the impact that we were hoping for. In fact, adding and removing color can have a detrimental impact on the hair. Instead of achieving that glossy look we were striving for us all too often end up with dull, lifeless looking hair.

Chapter 7:
Essential Makeup Strategies

Makeup can work miracles to cover your flaws and enhance your beauty quotient. But, if you go too overboard with the makeup, you may end up looking like a mannequin. To ensure you do not look all caked up, natural makeup methods can be of significant help.

When you talk of makeup, you can think of having the right look without using a foundation and a concealer. One great reason for your cake up look is when you make unwarranted use of either of the concealer or the makeup. If you want to have a very natural appeal and look, you must make minimum use of the concealer and foundation. It is similarly vital to pay close attention to the way you apply your foundation. To get the right look, ensure that you spread it evenly on the whole face.

Opt for a colored moisturizer rather than a regular one as they tend to blend in more evenly with the skin. Apart from having great moisturizing properties, it might also make your foundation unnoticeable to the naked eye. If you suffer from darker scars or blemishes, you may have to employ a concealer a bit more to cover them up. Do choose one that matches your skin tone to prevent the makeup from looking too artificial.

Your eyes demand absolute focus when you are working on your makeup. Use clear mascara to make your eye makeup appear natural. This will make your lashes look longer without making you look too over the top. Also, dab a bit of foundation on the eyelids too, as this may help even out the complexion.

When using an eyeshadow go in for lighter and fragile tones like bronze, orange, copper, or pale pink. Don't go in for extreme shades like blue or green as you would like to keep the look natural. Do not dab the eye shade too much. For the eyeliner too, avoid warped shades. Brown and charcoal gray work the best as they help give you a natural look. Mix them with the eye shade to form a natural line.

The lips are also important when applying makeup. To make your lips look natural as well as irresistible, refrain from using deep color shades such as brown or maroon. Super glossy or glittery lipsticks should also be avoided if you want a more natural look for yourself. Determine which shade will look most natural on your lips by biting them and checking the color that fills the spot. The shade of your lipstick has to be of the same. Once you have applied the lipstick, seal it with clear lip gloss to make it last longer. Otherwise, you could try and apply only transparent gloss to retain a pleasant appearance.

With these natural makeup techniques at your aid, you will be ready to s polish your face and still look at your natural best.

To look more appealing, others also tend to trim their facial lines. Some tips to do so effectively;

1. Choose the right shape for your eyebrow.

Your eyebrows play a key role in shaping facial contours. They should be substantial, not thick, with a defined bow in the middle. Arched eyebrows can lift the face. It may make the face look slimmer. Your eyebrows can stand out with eyeshadow a little darker than the color of your natural eyebrow.

2. Cover eye circles.

Eye circles affect how you look. You can cover them with concealer or a little white eye shadow, which can highlight the inside and outside corners of your eyes.Therefore, they help your eyes stand out. Your face looks slimmer when your eyes are highlighted in a good way instead of eye circles.

3. Blush placement as an experiment.

A little blush can make one look in pink. However, blush with red undertone can make the face heavier that it is. Apply it from the cheekbones to each ear in the middle. To avoid looking like a clown, just apply it lightly.

4. Play up eyes.

The more you play up your eyes, the slimmer you look. People won't focus on other parts of your face when their attention is drawn by your beautiful eyes. Your eyes appear larger with eyeliner and mascara. Eye shadow can work well with your eye color and the skin tone and. Blue eyes look charming with golden or pink eye shadow; green eyes look great with bronze and purple eye shadow; while blue, cyan and purple set brown eyes off to its advantage.

5. Apply bronzer correctly.

Your face can look slimmer if one uses bronzer correctly. Apply a light layer of bronzer. This application should be on the line of the jaw. The purpose is to darken the area slightly. Remember to blend it into your makeup. This is to avoid looking like a person with long beards. A light layer of bronzer applied under the jaw can draw the eye away from any fleshy part below your neck, but also can let you look 10 pounds lighter.

Chapter 8: Natural Facial Mask

As we all know, beauty is more than skin-deep. A glowing, smooth and acne-free skin is a desire of every person. To keep your skin healthy and free from acne and blemishes, you must be regular with your skin care routine and also follow healthy habits. Treating your skin with natural remedies has a universal appeal as they are free of any chemicals and harmful substances, thus causing no side effects. No doubt, the market is full of artificial skin care products, they are not only expensive, but can damage the skin in the long run. This is why it is more practical to opt for natural face masks and homemade skin recipes instead.

Applying face masks is an excellent way to rejuvenate the skin, deep clean the skin, exfoliate skin, extract dirt and grime from deep within the pores, remove blackheads and whiteheads in a safe and natural way to get a radiant glow. Some of the beauty experts recommend that facial mask should be used at least once a week. Facial masks can be energizing, soothing and help your skin to retain moisture. The main purpose of a facial mask is to nourish the skin to make it full of life, to get away from usual aging and dullness. They can draw blood to the skin's surface which further enable the stimulation of blood circulation. As a result, the skin gets moisturized, stabilized, preventing it from aging and drying, and even skin illnesses and irritations are prevented and treated.

The biggest benefit of natural face masks is that they are available in a large variety regardless of a person's skin type. However, whether an individual has an oily skin, dry or a combination of both, they can get the face masks suiting their skin type. Those who are sensitive to commercial mask ingredients can make their natural face mask with some foods like oats, avocado, banana, strawberries, tomato, cucumber, honey, blueberries and many more. They are powerful ingredients which contain natural vitamins and minerals. They can penetrate deeper and beneath the skin layers. They nourish the skin deeply. While using masks, make sure that they are properly absorbed by the skin. Some of the best all-natural ingredients for a natural hydrating face mask are Natural Vitamin E, Avocado Oil, and honey. Not to mention that these ingredients have anti-aging qualities as well as are very nourishing for all skin types.

Just before applying the treatment, you can give your face a soft massage. Make sure that all masks should be applied to a freshly washed face, rinsed with lukewarm water. Warm water helps in opening the pores and maximizes the treatments effectiveness. This leaves younger, tighter skin, healthier cells exposed with a more glowing complexion. It will also reduce the fine lines and wrinkles around eyes and lips. When used once in a month, the effective results can be seen, and a person could maintain a more youthful look.

While it's not unheard of for men to try natural face masks to better their skin, women are hands down the main admirers of this apparently ageless tradition. Look in the skin care section of any store and you're likely to notice a lot of different face masks that come in a variety of varieties. Numerous are set for on the spot use while some might need to be blended with water to start with. You'll also notice the cost of face masks may vary significantly, and this itself often causes people to make choices which might be far from being perfect.

Unfortunately, inside the makeup products industry, a higher price doesn't constantly equal higher quality. In reality, even many of the most high-priced cosmetic products you find on the shelves will result in a certain amount of harm to your skin. Several high-street brand names consist of fillers. These are substances which are usually added so as to make up the base of a product, as well as to create bulk. Most of the time, the filler will have petroleum based ingredients, some form of alcohol, together with a selection of several other chemicals, like chemical preservatives, etc.

Natural face masks should contain virtually no chemical substances whatsoever.However, attempting to locate such face masks in the average shop is virtually impossible. This, in turn, has essentially been responsible for the resurgence of homemade face masks, and in contrast to what many people assume, producing the face masks is exceedingly easy. Do-it-yourself face masks also can help you save a reasonable amount, depending on how lavish you would like to be.

One very basic mask necessitates absolutely nothing besides honey and oatmeal. First your oatmeal is simply put through a kitchen food processor or possibly a regular coffee grinder. Honey will then be combined with creating a pleasing rich paste that may be applied to your facial area at night just after you've had a bath or shower. Leave your mask on for 15 to 20 minutes. Then rinse it off. This will leave the skin looking glorious and healthful, and it'll likewise make sure the skin is sufficiently moisturized.

Working with some fruits as well as vegetables with your face masks is also a fantastic way to beat the signs of aging. Quite a few traditional labels do of course possess some fruit extracts, nevertheless, as you can certainly imagine, these types of extracts can't compete with the real thing. There's also a plethora of essential oils you can add to face masks, like tea tree oil, lavender oil, rosemary oil, to name only a few.

When buying your essential oils, always be sure to obtain those that are cold pressed simply because some extraction treatments eliminate much of the original goodness, and in some cases, the oils can, in fact, change from being very good for skin to being unhealthy for the skin. There are so many tested recipes around, we could by no means hope to go over them in such a small write-up, and so if you're seriously interested in creating your anti-aging masks, just perform some online research concerning the different ingredients you'll have to have.

However, should your routine doesn't let you produce your natural face masks, or maybe you believe you just don't want to, there are many fantastic products out there, nevertheless it's going to demand a little bit of research on your part

Chapter 9:
Natural Mask Recipes

Tea Tree Mask - The first of the recipes for masks for pimples uses oil from a tea tree. This oil, which is a completely natural remedy for pimples. It works as well as the benzoyl peroxide which is well-known, but doesn't have the bad side effects that peroxide different ways, including masks, toners, and spot treatments. Most people look for facial mask recipes because they kill off the bacteria that cause acne and heals the acne blemishes that are active. To make this first of the recipe for combining three drops of the oil with a mud mask that is pure clay. Mix this thoroughly and then put it on your skin. Once it's dry (it takes around 10-15 minutes), rinse your face well with some warm water.

Baking Soda - This second of the recipes for the masks for pimples uses baking soda. It is alkaline. As a result, it is helpful for killing the Candida bacteria. This bacteria may cause acne. Not forget that acne is usually resistant to treatment. You can use the soda as an exfoliant, a mask, or a tonic. Combine a teaspoon of baking soda with two tablespoons of mud mask that is pure clay and put it on your face. Leave your mask on for up to 10 minutes, and then use warm water to rinse your face off.

Oatmeal Mask - This is very soothing and when it's put on the skin can help with alleviating the inflammation and irritation that comes with acne. It's also possible to mix up this one of the recipes for masks for pimples is to use after you use another treatment for acne. It will help with soothing the skin and preventing acne breakouts from irritation. Combine half a cup of ground oatmeal with a quarter cup of hot water. Allow your mixture to cool, and then put it on your face. After a quarter an hour, rinse the mixture from your face with warm water.

When you are looking for recipes for masks for pimples, you are going to find that there are a lot of different choices. You will find hundreds of recipes on the web, and you can choose the one that is best for your type of skin. The three recipes for masks that are listed above are just a start for the plethora of different facial masks that you can choose from. Have fun looking for them and experimenting with them.

Are you fed up with spending so much profit in a spa and then let someone let you know the skin is awful? Well, don't worry. There are numerous items in your kitchen which work just like should you have had a day in the spa. This is more economical since you're using things you normally find in your kitchen countertops - bananas, vinegar, lemon, egg, milk, oatmeal, yogurt, mayonnaise, and mustard. Here are a few simple tips for making an excellent facial mask from these cheap ingredients.

- Banana. Bananas contain a lot of nutrients that may leave your skin moisturized. That's right! So who needs Botox if you have this fruit as a substitute? All you need to do is mash a ripe banana right into a smooth, soft paste. After which you can apply it to your neck and face. Set it for 10-20 minutes before you rinse it. You may also add other ingredients, for example, yogurt and honey to make a different type of mask.

- Egg. For any little bit of pampering of the epidermis, go and grab an egg. This breakfast favorite comes complete with nutrients which are great for your skin; as a result, it's a facial mask staple. For those who have dried-out skin, you simply need the egg yolk to do something as a moisturizer. The egg white is good for those individuals who've oily skin. You can include a bit of lemon or honey. Lemon and honey will strengthen the effects. Beat the entire egg to make your mask when you have normal skin. Just wait for 30 minutes before you rinse the residue.

- Vinegar. Vinegar is proven to be the most effective skin toner because the medieval period. Just add a tablespoon of apple cider vinegar to 2 cups water and put it on to your face after washing it. This helps your skin and then minimize your pores.

- Lemon. This citrus fruit can act as a great moisturizer and exfoliates your skin perfectly. Just add the juice of the fruit to some bit of olive or sweet almond oil for an excellent moisturizing facial mask.

- Milk. Milk is not only great for the bones and teeth; for milk is also a great source to have supple skin. Just mix powdered milk and water to create a paste before coating it onto your face. After which you can rinse them back with warm water.

- Mustard. You wouldn't imagine that mustard, a well-known hot dog condiment, can be an effective facial mask. This yellow substance helps to instimulate and soothe the skin.However, ensure you test on a small area before you apply it on the face.

- Oatmeal. Make your oatmeal facial. Just combine warm water and oatmeal together and watch for it to settle down. After it settles, mix in some yogurt, honey and egg white for an all-natural facial mask.

- Yogurt. If you want to minimize your pores, that can be done by getting a yogurt facial. Yogurt helps tighten pores and cleanse your skin to provide you with that revitalizing glow. You may also add some orange juice and aloe to provide you with a more supple looking skin.

- Mayonnaise. Who says mayonnaise is just used as salad dressings? Surprisingly, they are just like any facial creams you have in your cabinet. Add a whole egg with this ingredient and you'll possess a smoother and cleaner face in a few minutes.

Chapter 10:
Some Organic Beauty Treats

Some of the natural beauty recipes and ingredients that have proven useful are:

- Body scrub ingredients for exfoliating

- Body scrub ingredients for moisturizing

- Body scrub ingredients for moisturizing

- Body scrub ingredients for perfume

Body scrub ingredients for fragrance.

Add aromatherapy oil, just a drop or two. This is indeed the perfect addition. Lavender is relaxing, eucalyptus and citrus are invigorating. Experiment and choose your favorite.

Mixing the body scrub ingredients to put the dry exfoliating ingredients.

- Include a little oil, just bit by bit. This should be until you develop a creamy enough taste to spread like an ointment around on your skin.

- Give a drop of your favorite fragrant oil and mix it in thoroughly.

- Now enjoy the home treatment of healthy spa, or package your homemade present in an appealing container.

One can generate their recipes by understanding how effortless they are to make. Also, one should understand how great they make one feel.

Sensitive skin exfoliation mask

If you would like a gentle skin exfoliation, then try our unique recipe, one that you may not find anywhere else. First get a bowl and mix a cup of cornmeal, a cup of milk, two teaspoons baking soda, one tablespoon olive oil and five drops of tea tree oil to make a kind of paste. Apply this to your skin and leave it to set for around 15 minutes. After 15 minutes you can start taking it off with a muslin facial cloth as this will gently exfoliate your skin rather than just washing off the solution.

Sea salt exfoliation scrub.

Sea salt has been one of the most natural exfoliation products available for generations now. You can buy this from various shops, and one tub can last you up to 12 months as all you need a pinch or around one teaspoon of the salt. You then apply it to your entire face and exfoliate using your fingertips. You should be able to feel the salt working away on your skin.

Ever used homemade soap?

Ever thought of making your soap? Well, now you can. Nothing is more luxurious and relaxing than a block of shear butter soap gliding on your skin before you say good night.

Some simple ingredients that you will need to make the soap: Castile soap (olive oil based), distilled water, 2 tablespoons of unprocessed Shea butter, 1 tablespoon finely ground almonds (this is an optional ingredient), a grater to grate the almonds, 1 small pot, 1 big pot, a small plastic food container, a mixing spoon and drying rack.

Once we have the necessary equipment and ingredients ready to use, we can put the water to boil in the big pot. While the water is boiling, we can grate the Castile soap, this grated powder should fill 2 cups. The grated powder can then go into the small pot, which can then go into the pot of boiling water to allow the soap to melt. Keep stirring the mixture, only stop when the soap feels stringy and tight as you try to remove the spoon from the mixture.

Once it has melted and gone to a like stringy structure, feeling a bit of stickiness as you try to remove the spoon, you can take it off the heat and start adding the remaining ingredients such as the Shea butter and almonds. Once you have got these final ingredients to blend in nicely, we recommend placing the blended mixture in a plastic container, to allow it to set into like a cube or rectangular structure. Once it has set in the container, remove it and allow it to dry on the drying rack, please give it three weeks to settle, keep rotating to avoid getting grid imprints from the rack on the soap. The soap can then be wrapped in a plastic wallet, ready for use during your next bath or shower.

Wrinkle smoothing recipe.

You can start saving some money on your beauty regime by using our extremely budget banana recipe. Banana is extremely good to remove wrinkles and moisturize the skin. All you need is bananas, mash into a paste and apply it on the skin. While it's working its magic on your skin for 15 minutes, you can enjoy eating the other half of the banana. After 15 minutes, wash your face with warm water. You can then-then add a splash of cold water at the end to close your pores.

Chapter 11:
Maintain The Look

Phthalates (pronounced "Thal-rates") are a little harder to spot than other toxic beauty ingredients. This is because they are usually found within a fragrance and aren't listed separately. It takes extra legwork to find out whether or not a store-bought product contains phthalates. Why should you bother to keep an eye out for phthalates? Like parabens, phthalates have possible connections to reproductive toxicity and endocrine disruption. They are also linked to developmental issues, making their safety questionable for pregnant women, nursing moms, kids, babies, and pretty much everyone else.

CUSTOMIZE YOUR RECIPES

As you replace products from your routine, you'll start to notice what does and doesn't work for you. Is your skin dry? Is your hair heavier or oilier than you'd like? Many of the everyday recipes in this book contain information on customization and troubleshooting. Once your routine is established, it's a good idea to take a close look at each segment and make any necessary adjustments.

If you have a condition such as eczema, psoriasis, or chronic dry skin, pay extra attention to how your skin reacts to new recipes, ingredients, or changes to your routine. If you are under a doctor or dermatologist's care, discuss your natural beauty plan with them before you get started.

KEEP IT SIMPLE

If you do a little searching, you can dig up plenty of recipe books for natural beauty. The biggest difference between this book and many other natural beauty books is that the recipes in this book are given in their most simplified form. While experimenting with exotic ingredients and complex formulas can be fun, keeping things simple is the best strategy for establishing an everyday routine.

Everyday skin care and hair care is similar to everyday cooking and eating. The healthiest options often depend on simple combinations of high-quality ingredients. Quality over quantity matters. For example, a great facial oil doesn't have to contain twenty different ingredients: Just one or two that work well will suffice.

FRESH IS BEST

Commercial beauty products have been formulated by scientists to remain shelf table. Mass produced recipes won't go bad before their expiration date and are built to withstand direct handling and less than ideal storage. Handmade products don't have the protection of high-powered preservatives so keeping them fresh depends on proper storing and handling.

We aren't used to thinking of beauty products in the same way that we do food but, the truth is, they are often made from the very similar stuff. You wouldn't want to eat a meal that has been left on the kitchen counter overnight, and a fresh batch of the handmade lotion is very much the same. The best way to safely use homemade products is to make them to order. Create products in small batches, use them up quickly, and always try to handle products and ingredients with clean hands.

DEVELOP A ROUTINE

Sometimes you have to kiss a few frogs before you find your Prince Charming. Falling in love with your natural beauty routine could take a little bit of trial and error as well. Not every recipe or technique will work for you right away. Sometimes it takes a little tweaking and a lot of practice to get something to work for you. Other times, you may find that you need a different method altogether. As you try different recipes and new ingredients, take note of how your skin and hair react. By continuing to make adjustments along the way, you'll end up creating a routine that is fully customized to your unique needs.

TOXIC BEAUTY INGREDIENTS

If you look at the label on store-bought shampoo, body wash or bar soap, you are likely to see an ingredient containing the word sulfate. Sulfates are types of detergents and surfactants that help create that rich, bubbly lather that we all love. Unfortunately, they also have a habit of stripping the skin of the beneficial oils that keep it moisturized and protected.

People with sensitive skin sometimes have very strong reactions to sulfates. Reactions can result in redness, rashes, and, in extreme cases, bleeding. Sodium Laureth Sulfate (also referred to as SLS) is a common sulfate found in bath and body products. It is one of the many sulfate ingredients that can wreak havoc on your skin and scalp.

Most natural beauty recipes are very easy to make. The sugar scrub above can be made by mixing just two ingredients—sugar and oil.

To establish a natural beauty routine that works you need to do four things:

Give each recipe, ingredient, or method a fair shot. Your skin needs time to adjust any time you change a routine. It's important to let that adjustment happen before you decide whether or not something works for you. As a general rule, it's good to give any change about seven days to settle in.

If your skin or hair has an extreme reaction or has an allergic reaction to an ingredient, stop using it right away. Instead, consider consulting a doctor.

Pay attention to your body. Your skin and hair have a way of telling you what they need. Paying close attention to how your body reacts to the recipes you use can help clue you into how they can be adjusted to suit better your needs.

The recipes in this book can be used as-is, but are far more effective when customized to a specific skin type or hair type. No two people are the same, which can make customizing recipes a challenge. When it comes to establishing your routine, you are the best possible person for the job. Find a balance that works for you. When it comes to natural beauty, it's not all or nothing. Some people like to keep their hair care all-natural, but aren't ready to give up their favorite facial cream or commercial deodorant. That's okay! The two Worlds don't have to be mutually exclusive.

Any changes you choose to make will be worthwhile. While there are certain recipes that need to be used together (and I'll point those out as they come along), usually you can pick and choose which portions of your routine to keep all-natural. For example, you might choose to

Cleanse and condition your hair naturally, but continue to style your hair with commercial gel.

Be consistent. The recipes in this book are meant to help you create a whole new way of caring for your skin and hair. Repeatedly switching back and forth between handmade and commercial products is likely to wreak havoc—especially for those methods that involve a long adjustment period. Do yourself a favor, and do your best not to "cheat" on your natural routine.

Conclusion

Keeping your good looks is very important in today's world. People are making their first impressions quicker and quicker, so you need to really stay on top of things. To make matters worse, it's easier than ever today to lose sight of things and to make it difficult to maintain your beauty, both your natural internal beauty and the external beauty that you work so hard to maintain.

When you meet somebody for the first time, you obviously want to look your best. This is like working out. You have to work hard to stay in good shape, but a few bad habits can ruin everything. And the sad thing is that in today's society bad habits are easier than ever to pick up, and harder than ever to get rid of.

We live on a planet that provides us with everything we need to be well, bright and beautiful. In some cases, though, our intellect simply has not led us to find the plants or minerals which hold our cures. Even as we speak, scientists are investigating corals from deep on the ocean floor and their effects on pancreatic cancer.

Minerals have become the stuff of opulent skin creams and the latest craze. And yet, they were always there. Our knowledge just had to catch up with them. As our illnesses and social diseases change so will plant and minerals continue to evolve to counteract their effects. There is such a feeling of satisfaction, I find, in making my products at home.

I am sure you will be thrilled too when you discover how adapting recipes for your skin works so very easily. Please don't take my word for it. Get out there in the garden and find dandelions and roses. Substitute an oil here for a smidgen of crystal there. Make it up, mix it up... have fun!

Beauty comes in all shapes and sizes. Perhaps it's the part of a woman which never quite dies. Most assuredly it is the passion in the things which give her great joy. Whether that's her garden, her children, or making her pots of cream. You'll never know if this sparks that glint of magic in your eye unless you try it

The first thing is not brushing your teeth correctly. Many people just load up their toothbrush with some toothpaste, and just go to work for a few minutes and think that's good enough. However, if you don't floss, you are leaving the gaps between your teeth filled up with ugly gunk. This can look terrible when you smile, so please take the time not only to brush thoroughly but to floss as well.

Another thing that can cause some serious negative effects when it comes to beauty is picking at acne. This can be incredibly hard to resist, but resist you must. If you keep picking at your acne, this will cause scars later on. And if you have scars, no amount of makeup can cover this up. You might look good from a few feet away, but when people get close to you, they'll notice all of the acne scars. Then they'll only be able to think of you as a pimply kid, instead of a professional adult.

If you don't drink enough water, your skin can easily dry out. Most people only drink when they are thirsty, but this is already too late. You've got to drink plenty of water. This should be done possibly throughout the day. If you don't, your skin will be dry and will age prematurely. You might not be worried about this now, but when you hit forty or fifty years old, you'll wish you had hydrated more often.

Avoiding these habits will go a long way in keeping you looking young and beautiful. Because that's very important, you should avoid these habits at all costs.

Thank you for taking your time in joining me as we explore this journey of beauty. It takes a whole more than just a one-time dressing and makeup. Beauty is a lifestyle and once properly embraced makes to be at a new level of life.

I believe this book has been informative for you so far. Please leave a review for this book. This is to help me as the author knows to what extend this writing has impacted on you as the reader.

www.ingramcontent.com/pod-product-compliance
Lightning Source LLC
Chambersburg PA
CBHW071253280526
45788CB00004B/1703

9 781530 246120